Thin (Inside)
A Handbook for the Understanding of Weight-Challenged Individuals

By Paolo Mancini

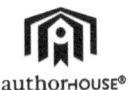

authorHOUSE®

AuthorHouse™
1663 Liberty Drive, Suite 200
Bloomington, IN 47403
www.authorhouse.com
Phone: 1-800-839-8640

First published by AuthorHouse 1/16/2009

ISBN: 978-1-4389-3656-7 (sc)

Library of Congress Control Number: 2008911026

Printed in the United States of America
Bloomington, Indiana

This book is printed on acid-free paper.

Cover Design by Zerostreet Studios
www.zerostreet.com

Cover photograph "Untitled Vase" courtesy of Armando DeJesus

For more information about the author visit his website at
www.paolomancini.com

Dedication

I dedicate this book to my family. They have always supported me and loved me, thick or thin: my mom, Gladys; my father, Giovanni; and my brothers—Giovanni Jr., Pierluigi, Aldo, and Fabrizio—and their families.

And to my loved ones and friends, for they have always believed in me, and accepted me regardless of my weight: John, Junior, and Kelly.

Thank you.

Table of Contents

Chapter Zero

Introductions Are in Order.

Yes. In my magical world, there is such a thing as "Chapter Zero." Join me, if you will, on this journey I am calling **Thin (Inside)**.

By the way, in case anyone is wondering, we have reached the point in which the twenty-first century is well on its way. I have chosen to begin this book with these words because I stand in amazement as to how we continue, as a society, to view and deal with the issue of weight.

Theoretically, we have been made to believe that throughout history, people are supposed to continuously get better and smarter; and yet, society continues to feel compelled to pursue this insatiable quest for the perfect body, the perfect abs, the perfect buns, and the overall illusion of the perfect look—whatever that may be *today*. And believe me, that illusion changes all of the time—just take a look at your parents' high school yearbook if you don't believe me.

We live in a society where the infomercial and "reality" weight-loss programs rule, the exercise machines and gym memberships sell, and books about diets and weight loss programs abound—many of them turning out to be best sellers!

To me, it seems that in the quest for physical success, we have forgotten to attempt to understand the life, thoughts, emotions, and challenges faced by the so-called "weight-challenged" individuals on a daily basis.

Weight-challenged is the politically correct word for what the average person refers to as *fat.* Don't get me wrong; I'm not necessarily happy being fat, even though some people may very well be. And as long as there are no health problems (or risks) involved for that individual, I say there is nothing wrong with being, do I dare say it, chunky.

But for others, as well as for me, being fat is simply a reality that is very tough to change—a reality that chips away at our self-esteem and a reality that I am sure will excite the many doctors, psychologists, and so-called "experts" awaiting my phone call for a full analysis and weight loss program.

Well, guess what? *I don't need fixing.*

I need time, acceptance, and an understanding environment that allows for proper education of food, exercise, and the emotional reasons behind how we view both.

Unfortunately, we live in the real world, and thus I am forced to write this book (handbook, really) so that we, as a society, can all understand fat people: where we are at, where we are heading, and most importantly, what our main obstacles are. I hope you enjoy...

Thin (Inside)

A Handbook for the Understanding of Weight-Challenged Individuals.

On a side note, please understand that all of the comments mentioned in this book are just my own personal opinions. I am not a doctor, psychologist, or health expert (nor do I pretend to be one.) I am just an average person who speaks of his own experiences as one who is also *weight-challenged.*

Chapter 1

Why Am I Weight-Challenged?

Oh, okay, so there is no such thing as *weight-challenged. I am fat,* and I admit it. The only challenge I have is whether to "super-size it," "go-large it," "extra-size it," "value-size it," or "biggie it."

Actually, it is not much of a challenge when the answer is "All of the above, please, *and yes,* I do want some fries and dessert with that."

So what is the solution? Actually, there may not be one. Experts say a challenge is "an opportunity waiting to be defeated." I say a challenge is eating twenty-five Dunkin' Donuts Munchkins before getting home so that your family doesn't find out you are cheating on your diet. *Now, that's a challenge!*

But seriously, losing weight is definitely a challenge—a challenge that millions of honest and caring people in the world deal with every day.

I almost compare it to being addicted to alcohol. It is similar in that it does follow the same philosophy of "one day at a time," every day! The only difference, and it is a big difference, is that eating is not only *allowed, but a necessary part of life.*

This is the tricky part that makes controlling your diet really, really hard. How do you tell an alcoholic that he must stop drinking for his own benefit, but he can have only one beer a day? It wouldn't work. It would be like trying to eat just one potato chip. Impossible!

And this, my friends, is what makes this so challenging; for, you see, eating is a natural and necessary activity for our survival.

So is there a solution?

One solution I came up with in my journey is *not to think of it as a "challenge to lose weight," but to think of it as various small challenges within our daily lives.*

Here are some of the ones that I came up with:

(1) **Challenge yourself to learn as much as you can about the body you have.** Yes. That big, beautiful body your soul calls home. My basic response to people is that I'm fat because my soul required a five-bedroom home with a pool, a patio, and a two-car garage. The truth is that your body is your soul's temple or, as others may put it, "a well-oiled machine." And if it

is well maintained, it will last a long time. So make it a point to learn how your body works, what's good for it, what's bad, how much chlorine the pool needs, etc. Maybe it will make you think twice about what you eat. Which brings me to my second point...

(2) **Challenge yourself to learn more about what you eat on a daily basis.** Three key words represent the solution to this challenge: *read the labels*. Something that tastes great may get a second thought after you find out what's inside—chemicals, dyes, etc. You would be surprised to find out that some of your favorite foods or soft drinks can also be used to remove stains, polish silver, clean carpets, or remove unwanted rust.

(3) **Challenge yourself to listen to your body, legitimate experts only, and people who have travelled the same road.** You'll be amazed as to what your own body will tell you if you just stop to listen to it every once in a while. And be careful about listening to self-proclaimed experts. The diet industry is a multi-billion dollar industry, and everyone is out to make a quick buck. Don't fall for it. Follow the old, but wise, rule "If it seems too good to be true, it probably is."

(4) **Challenge yourself to learn about exercise.** Oh, no, that nasty and horrible word. Yup! I'll say it again: *learn about exercise.* Mind you, I didn't say "go to the gym." I said pick up a book and learn about exercise. Learn what type of exercise may be good and "fun" for you. I'll say this once: not every exercise is

good for everyone. And most importantly, *not everyone belongs in a gym* (we'll talk more about gyms later). There is, however, one honest truth, and that is that basic exercise does assist you in achieving your weight loss goals. Find out what exercise feels good to you and what exercise you may enjoy doing—and then, *enjoy doing it!*

(5) **Challenge yourself to understand your emotional body.** Yes. There are two types of bodies we need to be honest about and careful with: your physical body and, honestly, what I consider most important, your emotional body. Why do you eat? Do you eat when you are happy? When you are sad? When you are angry? When you feel lonely? Understand and pay attention to why and when you are eating, and you

will be surprised to discover emotional "triggers" that truly need to be dealt with. Most of these triggers do come from our childhood, so be willing to travel back and honestly let go of the past—and believe me when I say, I know "it's easier said than done." But if there is one thing I want you to learn from this book, it is that *no matter how much you diet and exercise, the weight will always come back if you do not deal with the emotional triggers that are making you overeat and may even make you feel more comfortable being fat.*

(6) This brings me to my sixth and final point. **Challenge yourself to have specific, detailed and realistic goals.** It is wise to make them small. The longest mile begins with only one small step. Don't try to become a body-builder in one day. As

a matter of fact, have a variety of goals: exercise, nutrition, emotional work, record keeping, etc. Keep in mind what I said earlier—a great goal needs to be specific, detailed, and realistic. And always start it with the knowledge that you are doing this "just one day at a time." And then ask yourself, *"How will I do today?"*

And those are the types of goals I try to set in my life. It's not easy, but it's not that hard either. Work slowly and methodically, and being *weight-challenged* may be a thing of the past, if you so desire.

Chapter 2

I Am Not a Model,
and I Don't Look Like One...Yet!

One of the worst influences that fat people must deal with most often today is the media. These wonderful tools of information—such as magazines, newspapers, television, the Internet, and the radio—are all constant reminders that being fat is pure evil and being thin and beautiful (and that's the tricky part, because just thin is not enough) is good and *necessary* to survive in this jungle we call life. *This is a lie.*

We are constantly reminded that if you don't look like a cover model in a magazine, *you do not exist.* What they don't tell you is that you are in the majority. Ninety-nine percent of the population of this earth would be considered by today's media as not meeting the requirements needed to be a beautiful person. And believe me when I say, *we are all beautiful.*

The other thing they don't tell you is that most of those cover models don't even look like that. One word: "airbrush." It means, in my dictionary, "a practice that enhances the illusion of something that is not real." And believe me, it is all an illusion. These models don't even look like that every day. And even though I agree that we should all look as good as possible (regardless of our weight), we may never look like that cover model. Repeat this aloud. "We may never look like that cover model." Again: "We may never look like that cover model." Accept this, repeat it often, and move on with your life.

Plus, what's so good about being what I would call "model-thin"? I do know that being a cover model is honest hard work, and may the almighty bless the few individuals that have what it takes to do this job. I mean, yes, there's the huge money, the fancy parties, the great clothes, the millions of people imagining you naked, wanting your body...wow! What was my point? Oh, yes: "We may never look like that cover model." Accept it, repeat it often, and move on with your life.

Even though now, I'm feeling a little sad. I wonder how late Burger King is open?

Which, I guess, brings me to my next point: *our emotions.*

Chapter 3

Is It All Just About Emotions?

Are you like me? Do you eat when you are happy? When you are sad? When you are angry? When you are stressed? I do. And if you are really like me, you realized that I missed the most important feeling of all: *eating when you are hungry.*

Fat people very rarely eat when we are hungry. You see, I'm *emotional* all day long, so I eat all day long and I very rarely get to experience being hungry. That is not a good thing!

Part of the problem—and I am speaking to those of us that experience on a daily basis the "emotional roller coaster" I call food—is that our way of thinking needs to change. At one point in our lives, we were taught that food was our *friend.* It can make us happy when we are sad; happy when we are angry; and even happier when we are happy. We use food as a "bridge" to an emotional state.

The sad part about this is that, because it is one of our learned triggers, this, for us, *does work.* Think of all of those people that get stressed out and go out and smoke a cigarette and come back feeling happy and relaxed. Now think about what a cigarette is. A cigarette, in my opinion, is an over-priced mixture of herbs and chemicals wrapped in a thin paper so that you can burn it and inhale its smoke.

What in the world is that?

It is all in the mind. The cigarette simply wakes up the emotional trigger that tells the individual that if they do this activity, they will go from a stressed state to a more relaxed or happy state.

This is why so may people continue to smoke while knowing all of the health risks associated with the habit.

They have not been able to find something else to manipulate their emotional state in such a way that can replace the cigarette.

And mind you, you can take the whole paragraph above and switch the word *cigarette* with *alcohol and drugs.*

And for me, a glazed Krispy Kreme doughnut may just be my cigarette. Everything from its first bite to its last (and sometimes it's the same bite) is wonderful. I feel like a happier person.

Mind you, *there is nothing wrong with eating a doughnut.* I'll repeat this. *There is nothing wrong with eating a doughnut.* You just shouldn't eat it just because you are sad, stressed, or lonely. You should eat it when you are hungry (and even then always in moderation).

This brings me to my next point: *diets and eating.*

Chapter 4

Diets: Friend or Foe?

I'll say this once: *all diets work*!* Actually, I think this is really important, so I'll say it again: *all diets work*!* What you may not have realized is that this statement has an asterisk (*) after it. This means, you've guessed it, a legal disclaimer (the fine print), which may read something like this:

All diets work*

*May involve some starvation, unnatural fasting, or malnourishment of your body. May involve removing important vitamins, minerals, and unnatural amounts of carbohydrates, sugars, and fat that your body may need to function properly. All results vary and are definitely not guaranteed. The people in our infomercial are paid actors, who may not have actually done our diet. Statements and pills not approved by the FDA. May cause dizziness, stomach cramps, uncontrollable diarrhea, an oily discharge, and other awful side effects. If not continued routinely throughout your entire life, all of the weight will come back in even greater amounts.

Now, I may have thought twice about starting that "diet" if I had read the fine print. And this brings me to my follow-up statement: *all "diets" fail.*

Diet is a word that has so many meanings, but a realistic meaning to me would be: "(step A) *a temporary change in eating routine to gain a desired weight level that can then* (step B) *be maintained through proper eating habits and regular exercise.*"

The question then would be, if the diet is just a temporary solution that without step B would not work, why not just skip the diet state altogether and just go to proper eating and regular exercise?

You'll be cutting out the middle man and much of the stress that comes from it. In other words, and these are my words of wisdom for the entire book, *learn to eat the way you'll eat the rest of your life.*

Why teach your body one thing if, when you get to your goal, you'll change the routine (and most likely go back to old, and probably bad, eating habits)? Once you have this down, stick to it and exercise regularly (fun exercise—and we'll talk about that later).

* The Price of Beauty *

I'll tell you honestly what one of my biggest problem is with diets and healthy eating in six words. *Fast food is so darn cheap!* When a salad (lettuce and tomato) costs as much as a bacon double cheeseburger, my mind tells me that the burger will fill me up more and give me more nutrition, and the sad part is that in most cases, the bacon double cheeseburger is cheaper than the salad.

Unfortunately, eating right seems to also be a financial commitment. Why pay almost $6.00 for a garden salad when a combo meal is $2.99? And that includes fries and a drink. *Who has that kind of money?*

Well, I have found a solution for this. I'm going to introduce a topic that may be scary to some of you: *cook at home.* Let's repeat it: *cook at home.*

You see, buying the food at your local super-market and making it yourself will cut the costs of eating healthy by more than half. Plus, you'll be sure that what you are eating is properly made, fresh, and made just the way you like it.

Not to say that fast food doesn't have a place in the world. Many a night I get home late and just don't feel like cooking, so a local burger or sub place is the perfect answer. We just need to be more careful with what we order on those occasions.

And to be honest, and I believe this to be true, you should reward yourself (every once in a blue moon) with that double burger and fries. It's important to realize that you should never completely remove something you like to eat (and I say *like* instead of *need;* please notice the difference) from your diet, If you do, you'll just end up frustrated and one day you'll explode and eat ten of whatever you have been depriving yourself of. The key is just having a small portion of it every once in a while—not too often. Like at the company pizza party, *one slice* and that's it. The key is to eat it slowly and enjoy every single delicious bite, knowing that you may not have it again for a while.

Chapter 5

Exercise, Training, and Other Evil Words.

We have gotten to the point of the book that the censors worried about. I told them I would say a dirty word in chapter five. Here it is: *exercise.* It's pure Evil with a capital E. It's no coincidence that it is spelled so similarly to "exorcise." You do the math!

Okay, okay, so exercise is not really a dirty (or evil) word; it's actually a necessary step to successfully losing weight.

For the sake of the censors, I will change the word "exercise" to "activity" in this chapter. For, you see, we may not want to exercise, but to do an activity with our friends may actually be fun. And that's the key—fun.

Don't get me wrong; the word *fun does* vary by the level and intensity of your activity and the program you place yourself in. At some point, those activities may be quite challenging, but this is also good. The old saying, "No pain, no gain" may apply, except for the fact that pain is not really a word we all want to experience.

How about changing that saying to *If you don't challenge yourself above and beyond the levels you are currently working on, you'll never gain results above and beyond the results you currently enjoy.* I guess that was too long for a bumper sticker, so they stuck to "No pain, no gain."

* Gyms *

This brings me to the one place everybody thinks they need to go as soon as they decide that they are overweight: the gym.

I have actually been there, to this strange place called a gym. It's fascinating. You actually pay someone money on a monthly basis to have to drive to this place to walk and lift things. Odd, but true.

Now, I'll say this once (from personal experience): if you are really heavy, the gym may not be for you. Yes, I said it. *The gym is not for everyone.* If you choose to go, and pay the monthly fee, you may soon realize that what you needed to start doing is an exercise (oops, activity) called walking.

Which, at the gym, you do in a fancy state-of-the-art machine called a treadmill. But guess what? The sidewalks of our neighborhoods are *free of charge.* Yes. It's true. Assuming you live in an area that is okay for you and a friend to go out walking (and if not, please do go to the gym and walk there—safety first), the sidewalks are an excellent place to walk with a friend.

Some fast walking for about maybe forty-five to sixty minutes each day (morning or afternoon) while you chat about this and that may be the fun activity you may have been looking for.

Just make sure you are walking fast enough to break a sweat. *Sweating is good.* And drink plenty of water so that you can keep your body hydrated.

If you do go to the gym to begin the process of losing weight, just get on the treadmill for about forty-five to sixty minutes each day and walk at a quick, but comfortable, pace. Measure the speed that your body is able to do, and then just increase it periodically.

Important note: whatever you do, at this stage, *avoid the trainers.* Trainers (and we will talk about them later) do have a place in developing your body (in the *instruction* phase). In the beginner's phase, all you need to do is just keep walking and losing fat until you feel comfortable with moving towards working out and toning your body.

Now, trainers will tell you that lifting weight creates muscle and muscle burns fat faster, and this is true. But keep in mind that you are a larger person wanting to lose weight—and this may be your first time in the gym. You want to take small steps so that you can acclimate yourself to the environment first. This is important because if you don't acclimate well because you are trying to do too much too soon, you may just stop going altogether—which is not working toward the goal.

* Wearing Your Gym Uniform *

Another issue, while we are at the beginner stage and probably at our heaviest: let's talk clothing. I'll say this once: *no leotards or stretchy material of any kind!*

Have you ever walked through a mall and seen pretty stores and then run into an area covered by wood panels which mentioned "Coming soon...xyz store"?

Well, that's you and your body. *We are under construction.* And an oversized, dark t-shirt and shorts (or sweatpants) are the appropriate clothing for this phase. Let us be that store which is preparing itself for the grand opening.

Also, and this comes back to clothing, when you are fat and in a gym, you are probably the minority.

Typically, people that go to the gym are people that find it enjoyable to work out (yes, they exist) and like to have their bodies on display to prove it. So, don't wear anything to draw attention to yourself. Dark, loose-fitting clothes are better. The reason I mention "not standing out" is that you may begin to start feeling self-conscious about your weight and may decide to stop working out altogether.

Not to mention the fact that you may have already paid the $300 non-refundable annual membership for a gym that you are no longer using.

Just go, do your walking, sweat, and go home. I would not even recommend taking a shower in the gym. You may get back to that self-conscious state if you see a person with a perfect body taking a shower next to you.

And believe me, the last thing you need when you "do activities" in the gym is to feel self-conscious about how you look like and what you are doing.

Your body is *under construction,* and with hard work and consistency, you will definitely unveil a tremendous grand opening to that beautiful store you now call your new body.

A key to a successful workout for beginners is to go with a friend. If you don't have one, go alone, and soon you'll probably notice another chubby person on the treadmills every day around the time you go and *make a friend.* And keep each other motivated to keep going. Make it a point to meet each morning and do the walking together. This will make it more like a fun activity than exercise. Soon after that, you'll find yourself working towards the next level...which brings me to my next subject, *the trainers.*

Chapter 6

Trainers and Communication.

Let's say you've gotten your body to a comfortable weight, and you want to start lifting weights and working out with the machines. It is now time to seek "the trainer."

Before I speak of my horrible stories, please note that there are very good trainers out there and people that truly care about your health and wellbeing—people that take their time, not just to make you work the machines in a "drill sergeant" manner, but to explain the why, the how, and the frequency at which you should use the machines so that you truly understand what each machine does and can effectively create a routine that works well for your body.

Trainers should be *educators* and not *baby-sitters*. And there are a lot of trainers that believe in educating their clients; unfortunately, none of the ones I have had the misfortune of meeting seemed to share this belief.

For, you see, "baby-sitting" is how my trainers made their money. If they don't really teach you how to use the machines (and what muscles you are working, and why it is important to work out that muscle, etc.), they make you rely on them for your routine during each of your workouts. This way, you find yourself needing to pay them, week after week, to do your routine until you run out of money and are left without knowing how to work out on your own.

At this point, you don't have the money to get a new trainer that would hopefully be an educator, and you can end up giving up on the whole idea of working out. It happened to me this way.

It's a sad cycle that I went through several times, each time making me more disappointed in trainers in general.

On the other hand, it is important to remember not to do the machines without a trained expert to show you how to use them properly. Each machine is actually quite complicated and very specific to a muscle group or body part. A hand placement or incorrect seat level could end up working a very different muscle from what you were intending to work, or even cause injury.

Trainers: *"you can't live with them; you can't live without them."*

* Communicate Your Needs *

The key to finding a good trainer is communication. Most trainers give you a free consultation so that they can "sell" themselves to you. And this is important to remember: *you are the one paying* with your hard-earned money during your expensive session. *They are working for you!*

Don't forget that. It's crucial. A trainer is quite an expense; this is why most trainers offer a free consultation. The key is, instead of them telling you during that time why you would be the perfect client for them, use that time and interview them so as to decide if they would be the perfect trainer for you. Communication is the key!

Tell the trainer specifically what you are looking for, not just for your body, but from your trainer. If you see the slightest bit of hesitation in them meeting your demands, walk away!

There are thousands of good trainers waiting to help you reach your goal.

And what should your demands be?

(1) **Punctuality.** If you say seven o'clock a.m., it does not mean seven-fifteen a.m.. Your time is valuable; make them respect that.

(2) **Instruction.** You do not want them to just supervise your workouts on the machines, but instruct you on questions like these:

    a. How do you use the machines properly?
    b. What muscles would you be working out with that particular machine?
    c. What should your position/posture be to work out those specific muscles?
    d. What should the repetitions be for the various levels of experience—beginner, intermediate, advanced?
    e. What should be the order in which you should use the machines for maximum results?
    f. How should you break up your workout so that you work a specific region on a specific day?

(3) Structured scheduling. Have them write you a schedule of your workout so that you can continue on your own after they are no longer assisting you.

(4) Follow-up. Explain to them that you may need assistance again as you change to a different level.

When you hire a trainer, *never hire someone for more than three weeks.* After three weeks, you should know the routine and be able to do it for yourself. Rather than hiring a trainer for nine weeks because you feel you won't be able to do the routine without the instructor pushing you and motivating you, just give your money to a worthy charity or organization and save yourself the hassle of working out. Why? Because you are not going to do it during that tenth and eleventh week, and you'll just end up never working out again. It's about self-motivation.

You must have the drive to work out on your own.

You can't rely on an instructor to motivate you, because when they are gone, you won't have somebody there to keep you going. And that's when the weight comes back.

A trainer is not just good for the first three weeks only. Let's say you learned the machines and your routine pretty well. A few months down the line, you'll notice muscles developing, and you may be interested in developing different muscles and/or changing your routine. What do you do? Call your trainer. Tell them what you want, and they'll help you to develop a different routine for you to help you move up to the next level. They may change the way you do the exercises. They may even change you from machines to free weights. And then, hire them for just another three weeks so that you can make sure you have it all down.

The most important thing to remember here is worth mentioning again: try not to see your trainer as your motivation, just your teacher. Changing your routine and moving levels will keep it fun and keep you looking good.

Now you can start wearing those *fitted* clothes and begin to show off your body.

Chapter 7

Work, Stress, and Other Challenges.

When a person breaks down his/her typical day, a few things should be included: work (obviously, we all need a roof over our heads), exercise (or fun activities), and relaxation.

You may not know this, but for a fat person, all of these three things bring forth one thing: *stress*.

Even though most of us can probably imagine how work and exercise can be stressful things for an overweight person (even though, in the long run, exercise will help you reduce stress), you may be wondering how relaxation can be stressful. Well, it can, if you are overweight. I'll explain with a little personal story.

Picture this. A man, a stressed fat man (whom you have the pleasure to call the author of this book), decides to do one of the most stress-free activities on earth for the first time in his life. He decides to get a massage at a very fancy spa.

Just think of it: soft music, aromatherapy, gentle (yet firm) hands massaging your muscles and removing every single bit of stress from your body.

Sounds great? It should. And yet, it didn't quite work this way. Many spas are geared for people who consistently attend them—i.e. physically fit, wealthy, confident individuals. Not necessarily yours truly (at that time).

* The Spa Session *

First, we began with the ever-embarrassing question-and-answer session regarding what muscles in my body I wanted massaged (i.e. where was I feeling most tense). We then moved to the ever-scary moment in which they showed me the cost of such tactical maneuvers. Yikes! But, we are relaxing, so it's worth it!

Then they took me to the men's locker room, showed me my locker, and proceeded to hand me a towel that is supposed to be one-size-fits-all, but basically just got to hide one of my butt cheeks while leaving the other one in plain sight as perhaps a constant reminder that I may not have needed those extra fries with that burger.

I then got to walk by people coming in and out of the locker room with one cheek poking out of my towel.

I was then asked to "jump" on top of the massage table while the masseuse just stood there, and while I was hoping that the towel would just hang on for just a few extra minutes. After realizing that I should have jumped on the table face down, but didn't, I get to experience the ever-magical moment of rolling over on a narrow table while maneuvering a small towel with one hand (not as easy as it sounds if you're over three hundred pounds).

And there I was, face down, sweating, with red cheeks (on my face that is), ready to relax.

The massage begins. And then it hit me, the fact that I could not relax while a strange person was touching my body. Fine time to realize this!

Then, the conversation started while I was trying to relax. "Where are you from?" "What do you do for a living?"

All the while, I just continued to pray that the towel (which was now just lying across my buttocks) stayed put.

Then, I heard the words that created the most challenging moment of all. "Please turn face up." What? That's how I started!

So again, I began the process of turning over on a table that is about twenty inches wide, while my waist is about fifty inches around—all while trying to keep the towel in place and not flash my private property to the unsuspecting masseuse.

I finally do it. By now, I was really sweating and red, and my stress level had soared to a new height. And then I remembered the price I paid for this privilege, which didn't really help the situation. Needless to say, I was far from being relaxed when I left.

It's similar to the kind of feeling you get (and fat people will relate) when you try to take a bath in a regular-sized bathtub. Not possible. Don't try it. Move on.

* In the workplace *

At work, there are a few tips (or basic things you need to know) to keep in mind if you are attempting to lose weight or if you have some fat coworkers who may need your sympathy:

(1) **Fat people get hungry around three p.m.** It's a law of nature. Don't fight it. It can't be done. Fat people get hungry at around three p.m. At this point, you will see them (or should I say "us"?) standing in front of the candy machine, measuring the frequency at which we have eaten a particular candy bar. We do like diversity in our choices.

(2) Most fat people (and women, for that matter) love chocolate. It's just nature. Don't fight it. It can't be done. If you are standing between a fat person or a woman and chocolate, please move out of the way for your own safety. We are really not responsible for our actions. Now, I don't mean to generalize all fat people, nor all women, but the majority I've met.

(3) Candy machines are *not* our friends. Not only do they remind us that we have to pay $1.25 for a craving that would cost fifty cents at the supermarket, but sometimes they tend to break down at the most inopportune times, like at our highest craving hour, three p.m. And sometimes, they break down *after* we insert our money and make a selection. *Now, this is really annoying.*

Chapter 8

Clothing Stores and Mannequins. Oh, How They Mock Us!

Regardless of whether you call it your body, your temple, or just your skin, we are all born with this thick thing that covers and protects our inside organs from just falling out all over the place. Nice thought, huh?

Of course, some of us have a thicker coat than others. Very few of us are identical—which means we are all different, and that's what makes us special and beautiful—regardless of our body size. After all, without fat people, thin people wouldn't know they are thin. So you see, *you do exist, and you do have a purpose.*

Now, as we already discussed, society and the media tell us that we must be thin to be happy. This may be true for some people, but for others, happiness is more than just how you look or your body size. Happiness is how you feel about yourself, how your loved ones feel about you, and that smile that comes to your face when you look in the mirror and know you are a good person.

But why is the size of your waist so important to society as a whole?

Not only that, but to add insult to injury, the image that the media and society want us to achieve is one that I would call "supermodel-thin" or "mannequin-thin." I've yet to see a mannequin in a store window that is about thirty or forty pounds overweight. Honestly, they typically look like a teenager with an eating disorder.

* Clothing Stores *

Speaking of mannequins, let's discuss the issue of clothing stores. As a fat person, I am very disappointed about the largest size most stores carry. As if all of us fall between a minimum and maximum size. It just doesn't work that way. I say, if this is how it's going to be, some stores should just have signs outside that read "No fat people allowed."

This would save us a lot of time that we spend inside thinking there will be a "magical" rack with our size on it.

Or better yet, the store should have a scale underneath the floor outside of the entrance. If you weigh more than a certain amount, an alarm should sound and say, *"Keep out."* Embarrassing, yes; but honest.

* Clothes *

Another topic related to clothes revolves around revealing, sexy, and skimpy clothes. This may include bikinis, thongs, tank shirts, running shorts, see-through blouses, short-shorts, etc. For the benefit of confused fat people everywhere (and I include myself in this), I personally believe we should create a law that prohibits the making of certain clothes above a particular size—the "Looks Good Size" (or LGS). This is the maximum size in which an outfit would look good on a person. The LGS should be the alarm that advises people, "Hey, your particular body size surpasses the LGS for this outfit; please try something more suitable."

You may not know how tough it is to go through life knowing that you can only shop at about 1% of all stores out there. And even tougher when you realize in that particular plus-size store, everything tends to cost more. If you don't believe me, check it out. A bathing suit for $56 (and they only have one print to choose from).

It's hard work being fat. With the time we spend walking around from store to store seeing if they have our size, I'm amazed that we don't become thinner.

One final thought on clothes. Could someone find the person that invented the one-size-fits-all outfit and give him/her a big slap? (Okay, not really; I don't condone violence.) But we all know that one size *fits only one size.*

The idea of a one-size-fits-all outfit is that if you are bigger, you won't mind a tight, uncomfortable outfit, and if you are smaller, you won't mind a larger, baggy outfit. It is false advertising, and I think it should be outlawed—especially since most chunky people fall for it. Be careful.

Thin (Inside)

Chapter 9

The Art of Having a Life.

So the question that many of you may have is, "Can we still lead comfortable, fulfilling lives while being fat?" The answer is *Yes!*

The type of life you lead is commonly related to the amount of self-confidence you have in yourself. Think of your body as a car. Some people have two-seater BMWs, and some have a big HUMMER. You see, the size of the car that a person drives has little to do with the quality of the car or the fact that the car is still primarily used simply to get from one place to another.

They are both high-quality cars; one may just be bigger than the other. And that is the key. You may have a bigger car as a body—perhaps a van, a station wagon, or even an SUV—but it can still be one heck of a car!

The first key to having a happy life is ensuring that basically, everything does not revolve around being fat. This topic should not dominate your conversations or your activity decisions—even if part of your life is going to the gym with the goal of losing weight. In this scenario, all you are doing is going to the gym to lose weight and get in shape, not because you are fat.

The word fat *should not exist in your new reality.*

You need to believe that you are not defined, judged, loved, or hated because of your body.

Even though this may be the sad reality of our society, it does not have to be yours.

The second key is to have friends. As we know, friends are chosen for their ability to enhance our lives, and this may come from people of all shapes, sizes, colors, etc.

But I will say this: if you do have the opportunity to pick your own friends (and of course you do), *pick active friends.*

I knew this guy whose friends were always very heavyset and not very active. I asked him why this was the case, and he told me that around them, he felt like the skinny one.

There was only one problem with that way of thinking: the fact that the activities of this particular group always revolved around food, eating, dining out, doing indoor activities that did not require much physical movement, etc. This is not good.

Perhaps this is why I make the suggestion of making friends that are active—because, most likely, the activities you plan as a group may end up revolving around being active—walking, exercising, riding a bike, etc.

Of course, each case is evaluated differently. I leave it to you good people to make the decisions of who your friends (or lovers) are. Just remember, if you want to lose weight and all your friends do is talk about eating, that is not helping you.

Worse than that, if all they talk about is how fat you are and how you should lose weight, they are not helping your self-confidence either.

So we must take the initiative and surround ourselves with only positive people who do not consistently bring up the fact that we may be heavier than what society considers normal, regardless of the activity we may be doing.

Speaking of going out, and again, I'll say this only once, *all activities with your friends do not have to revolve around food.*

This is very important.

Key places (or activities) to be careful with involve the magical sentence, "Hey, let's get together for lunch/dinner." This only leads to more body and less money.

Another place to be cautious (not avoid)—and this is one of my favorite places—is the movie theater.

Movies are designed to bring out emotions in us, not a good thing for people that eat based on emotions. Hot dogs, cheese nachos, anything chocolate, sodas, popcorn (with lots of butter, of course), etc. What was my point? Oh yeah, be careful at the movies. Always drink about two glasses of water before you go, and buy a bottle of water inside if you get cravings. If you must eat (and you are not allergic to them), sneak in some peanuts (not chocolate-covered). Be wise and be careful; you are really not allowed to bring food into a movie theater, so it would just be our little secret.

Clubs, bars, and discos are also tricky. Why? Emotions. In a club, you can get everything from nervous to happy to stressed to rejected. Be especially careful of those places that offer the free happy hour buffet. Another emotion you may experience in a social place like a club or bar is—well, how do I say this? — "lucky." And this brings me to my next point: *sex.*

Chapter 10

Sex with a Chunky Person.

It took me a while to decide whether or not to discuss this subject, and two reasons came up as to why I should:

1. I think it's important to see how sex is viewed by a heavier person, and

2. Come on, you must wonder about it when you see a heavier person. Admit it!

I'll speak from a guy's point of view on this subject, since I'm a guy. Ladies may find this way of thinking interesting too.

Why is sex a risky venture for heavier people? No, it's not the possible injuries that may occur (just teasing), but honestly, it's *emotions*.

When it comes to sex or "getting lucky," one may experience many emotions—happy (she wants me), sadness (she does not want me), confidence (she thinks I'm a god), doubt (she thinks I'm awful and nerdy), nervous (did I satisfy her?), and so on.

These emotions may culminate in the desire to overeat.

Remember:

> *Anytime you put yourself in a situation that may give way for an emotion to arise (which truly to some is their entire life), you have to be careful about those emotional triggers that may cause cravings for food.*

And speaking of triggers, I know as a guy, I'll move to a heavier person's second-biggest concern—size/satisfaction.

And by this, I do not mean your waist (this time). Not that size should matter, but I've always wondered if things would appear bigger with a smaller body. For those of you who may be wondering the same, let's look at this example:

Picture, if you will, a glass of water on top of a table. It looks a certain size and may look perfectly normal. Now imagine the same glass on top of a roof (from an aerial view). Does it look the same size (even though we know it is)? My conclusion after pondering this phenomenon was simple—I must lose weight now!

Now, sex in general with someone you care about and find attractive actually works the same for heavier and thinner people—*where there is a will, there is a way.*

For some, we just need to be a bit more creative than others; but I've always felt that this puts extra spice in the lasagna.

Did I just bring it back to food? Yes, I did. I just can't help myself.

And this brings me to my next point—*the reasons behind our cravings.*

Chapter 11

Why We Eat: My Theory!

Unfortunately, we cannot say that aliens from another planet came down and forced us to eat food through their hypnotic mind-manipulating powers. Even though that would make a cool program for the Food Network.

But seriously, think of food as fuel and your body as the car. You would never add more fuel to your car beyond the point at which you car says it is "full." Anything after that is just being spilled on the floor while you continue to pay between $3.00 and $4.00 per gallon (based on where you live). Gas is far too expensive.

So why would you give your body more food than what it needs to survive? Let's face it, even though I can (and have) eaten a dozen doughnuts in one sitting, my body didn't need that many. So I find myself not only paying for these extra doughnuts I didn't need, but spilling them inside my thighs and belly to carry around with me. Not a good idea.

A few personal theories about why we eat:
EMOTIONS

As we discussed earlier, I believe that emotional eating is what causes most of the overweight people in the world to be overweight. We do not properly deal with our emotions and simply believe we can make ourselves feel better by simply eating a cookie or a doughnut. The problem is that the feelings and issues do not go away, and you end up not only feeling depressed, but now, fatter!

FOOD ADDICTIONS

Guess what? Certain foods taste great. We need them. We crave them. We think we need to have them to survive (almost like a cigarette or alcohol). But the reality is that we can survive fine without them.

You would imagine that fat people eat everything and that's why they are fat, but the reality is that the fat people I know (including myself) are very picky eaters. We just eat a lot of the foods we like and for the wrong reasons (i.e. not just when we are hungry).

For example, I won't eat a salad, but give me a slice of pizza and you'll see the other seven slices disappear faster than you can say "pass the salad dressing."

The key to overcoming this is to allow yourself the pizza, but only the one slice. I believe that after a while, your stomach will shrink and that one slice will satisfy your craving and the need to eat the other seven slices will be gone.

NOTE: I want to make sure to stress how hard it is to control things like emotional eating or food addictions. These are issues that you may need external help with, like friends, family, and even a medical professional, if necessary. Just remember that you should only be eating when you are hungry (when the car needs fuel).

FINANCIAL RESOURCES

As we discussed earlier, non-healthy food costs less to buy than healthy food. A special message to all of the healthy food makers out there and to all of the fast food restaurants—*"Help us!"* My experience has been that it is truly cheaper, when eating out, to eat badly. Compare one dozen doughnuts for $2.99 versus a drive-through salad for $3.79. What will fill me up more? The mind will say "the doughnuts." And we know what the emotions will say. The key is to ask, "What is the better fuel to keep my car running smoothly in the long run?" And then the answer would be different.

* *Journaling* *

My only advice regarding the theory of why we eat is for you to keep a journal—just for three to five days (not a big project).

Write down all of the food you eat with a note on five things:

(1) What did you eat?

(2) When did you eat it?

(3) What emotion where you feeling before you ate it?

(4) Were you hungry before you ate it?

(5) And lastly, what was the reason you chose that food: emotional comfort, financial

cost, or "neither played a role—I just like it"?

And keep your normal eating habits; don't change them just because you are doing this assignment.

The goal of this is to slowly move yourself to only eat when you are hungry and to eat in moderation.

Again, I must emphasize that if you do find yourself eating mostly based on emotions, I would recommend seeing someone (a trained professional) to assist you in working those feelings out. If not, you may never be able to really curb that type of eating, and the weight will almost always come back.

Chapter 12

Holidays: Our Very Own Monthly Visitor.

This is a good place to speak about one of fat people's biggest enemies and a huge reason as to why we eat (or overeat). The answer lies in what I'd like to call the heavy person's monthly visitor—no, not PMS, but *holidays*.

It appears that there is a holiday almost every month of the year, and most of them revolve around food.

We have Thanksgiving, the Fourth of July, and Christmas (or Hanukkah or Kwanzaa), all revolving around a huge feast. We have Easter, Mother's Day, Valentine's Day, Halloween, all revolving around candy. We have St. Patrick's Day, New Year's, and the Super Bowl (not technically a holiday), revolving around food and alcohol.

It seems the only month that doesn't have a huge holiday is August, and that's my birthday month (August twenty-third, Virgo)—so you know there will be a birthday cake and a huge meal at my house.

Holidays are our enemies. I'll say it again: *Holidays are our enemies.* We must be very careful and stand firm around those times when our enemies attack. We must be strong and keep our will power intact.

There are three main things I would like to leave you with in regards to holidays:

It's okay to socialize without food.

This will be difficult, but social activities should not revolve around food, even though the people that create holidays would like for us to think so.

Eat only when you are hungry.

You'll be surprised as to how many times a day this actually happens. And yes, small meals often during the day will make our metabolism a continuous calorie-burning engine (continuing with our "body as a car" example.) And the goal is to get to know your body to a point that you'll be able to tell when your body's fuel tank is getting closer to "E" (empty) so that you can add some more fuel into it.

___Become more active during the holidays.___

Yes, this may include some exercise, but not necessarily. Go out more (and not just to dinners). Walk around the mall (it will keep you in tune with what is "cool" in today's world, especially if you have kids), play some golf, go to an art show and walk around, go to a craft fair and walk around, go to a museum and walk around—and believe it or not, you may even forget you are even "walking around"—but whatever you do, just go and do something.

Get your heart pumping and make new friends. Friends that understand (but won't bring up) personal challenges you may be facing with your body.

Trust me, this is important. They'll help you stay on course until you become more secure about what you are doing.

Chapter 13

The People We Love.

If there is one thing I've learned in life, it is that we cannot live happily without the people we love. Yes, the friends and family members that continuously keep repeating, "You would be so cute if only you could lose a few pounds." Ahhh, the sentence we have all heard. You do realize that they just basically called you ugly, right? Okay, just checking.

But what are we to do? It is those people that will love us even if we are fat, who will support us if we are attempting to lose weight, and who will be with us through thick (literally) and thin. Don't forget those people. Let them in.

I wrote this handbook as a guide for all of us to take a look at the world around us and laugh a little bit at what we see. So that people understand that we are all really thin...just some of us more on the *inside*.

About the Author

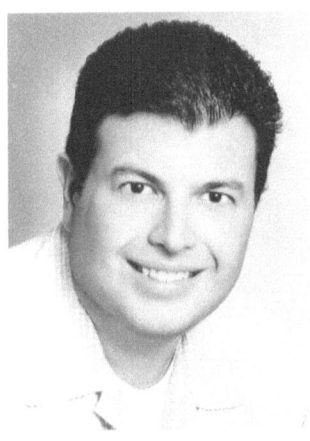

Paolo Mancini was born in Barranquilla, Colombia, and now lives in Atlanta, Georgia. **Thin (Inside)** is his first book. **Thin (Inside)** is the first book of a three part series which will include the soon to be published **Who Am I? (Inside)** and **Healing (Inside)**. He is also the radio host of METAmigoTalk, covering subjects related to metaphysics, spirituality, and the paranormal. For more information, visit his site at **www.paolomancini.com** or **www.metamigo.com** It has always been his belief that "without love, knowledge, and laughter, life would be a very sad and lonely journey."